Chrons Disease Cookbook

MAIN COURSE – 80 + Step-by-step recipes to improve gastrointestinal health and long-term wellness

TABLE OF CONTENTS

Introduction

Chrons Disease recipes for personal enjoyment but also for family enjoyment. You will love them for sure for how easy it is to prepare them.

BANANA AND APPLE PANCAKES

Serves: **3**

Prep Time: **5**   Minutes

Cook Time: **5**   Minutes

Total Time: **10**   Minutes

INGREDIENTS

- 1 apple
- 5 eggs
- 2 bananas
- 1 tablespoon coconut oil

DIRECTIONS

1. In a bowl mash the bananas and apples
2. Crack the eggs and mix them all together
3. In a frying pan pour one-two spoons of mixture
4. Cook each pancake for 1-2 minutes per side
5. Remove and serve with honey

Serves: *1*

Prep Time: *5*   Minutes

Cook Time: *5*   Minutes

Total Time: *10*   Minutes

INGREDIENTS

- 3 cups yogurt
- ½ cup almonds
- ¼ cup blueberries
- 1 cup strawberries
- ½ tsp lemon juice

DIRECTIONS

1. In a bowl place all ingredients
2. Mixed well and refrigerate overnight
3. Serve in the morning

Serves: *1*
Prep Time: *5*   Minutes

Cook Time: *5*   Minutes

Total Time: *10*   Minutes

INGREDIENTS

- ¼ cup oats
- ¼ cup milk
- ½ cup yogurt
- 1 tsp vanilla extract
- 1 tsp honey

DIRECTIONS

1. In a bowl combine all ingredients
2. Refrigerate overnight
3. Serve in the morning

Serves: *2*

Prep Time: *10*   Minutes

Cook Time: *10*   Minutes

Total Time: *20*   Minutes

INGREDIENTS

- 2 scrambled eggs
- 3 oz. salmon
- ½ avocado

DIRECTIONS

1. Scramble eggs and transfer to a plate
2. Add salmon, avocado slices and serve

Serves: **2**

Prep Time: **10** Minutes

Cook Time: **50** Minutes

Total Time: **60** Minutes

INGREDIENTS

- ½ tsp cinnamon
- 1 tsp canola oil
- 1 tablespoon oats
- 1 tsp sugar
- 2 apples

DIRECTIONS

1. Preheat the oven to 325 F
2. In a bowl mix sugar, cinnamon, oats and oil
3. Stuff into cored apples and bake for 40-50 minutes
4. Remove and serve

Serves: **2**

Prep Time: **5** Minutes

Cook Time: **10** Minutes

Total Time: **15** Minutes

INGREDIENTS

- 3 eggs
- ½ cup parsley
- ¼ tsp salt
- ¼ tsp ground pepper
- 1 tsp olive oil
- ¼ cup spinach
- 1 plum tomato
- ½ cup feta cheese
- 6 pitted Kalamata olives

DIRECTIONS

1. In a bowl whisk together eggs, parsley, pepper and salt
2. In a skillet add egg mixture and sprinkle remaining ingredients

3. Cook for 2-3 minutes per side

4. When ready, remove and serve

Serves: **2**
Prep Time: **10**   Minutes

Cook Time: **10**   Minutes

Total Time: **20**   Minutes

INGREDIENTS

- ½ cup peanut butter
- 2 bread slices
- 2 eggs
- ¼ cup almond milk
- 1 tsp vanilla extract
- 1 tablespoon sugar

DIRECTIONS

1. In a bowl whisk together eggs, vanilla extract, sugar and almond milk

2. Spread peanut butter over bread slices and top with bread slices

3. Dip each sandwich in egg mixture

4. Place sandwiches in a pan and cook for 5-6 minutes per side or until golden brown

5. When ready, remove and serve

ORANGE MUFFINS

Serves: **6**

Prep Time: **10**   Minutes

Cook Time: **20**   Minutes

Total Time: **30**   Minutes

INGREDIENTS

- 1 cup flour

- ¼ cup sugar

- 1 tsp baking powder

- ¼ tsp salt

- 2 eggs
- ¼ cup almond milk
- ½ cup butter
- 1 tsp grated orange rind

DIRECTIONS

1. Preheat oven to 375 F
2. In a bowl mix flour, sugar, salt and baking powder
3. Stir together almond, butter, eggs and dry ingredients and mix well
4. Spoon batter into muffin cups and bake for 18-20 ur until golden brown, remove and serve

BLUEBERRY MUFFINS

Serves: *4*

Prep Time: *10* Minutes

Cook Time: *20* Minutes

Total Time: *30* Minutes

INGREDIENTS

- 2 cups flour
- ½ cup sugar
- 1 tablespoon baking powder
- ¼ tsp salt
- 1 cup almond milk
- ½ cup butter
- 1 egg
- 1 cup blueberries
- 1 cup powdered sugar
- 1 tablespoon lemon juice

DIRECTIONS

1. Preheat the oven to 375 F
2. In a bowl place baking powder, salt, milk, butter and mix well
3. Stir together butter, milk and egg and mix well
4. Add dry ingredients, berries and mix again
5. Spoon batter into muffin cuts and bake for 18-20 minutes or until golden brown
6. When ready, remove and serve

Serves: *1*
Prep Time: *10*   Minutes

Cook Time: *10*   Minutes

Total Time: *20*   Minutes

INGREDIENTS

- 6 eggs
- ½ cup low fat milk
- ¼ tsp salt
- ¼ tsp pepper
- 1 tablespoon butter
- ½ cup cream cheese
- ½ cup Parmesan cheese

DIRECTIONS

1. In a bowl whisk together eggs, salt, milk and pepper
2. In a skillet pour egg mixture and sprinkle cream cheese and cook for 2-3 minutes per side
3. Remove and serve with parmesan cheese

Serves: **2**

Prep Time: **5**   Minutes

Cook Time: **25**   Minutes

Total Time: **30**   Minutes

INGREDIENTS

- **2 Tsp butter**
- **¼ shredded red cabbage**
- **5 eggs**
- **¼ Tsp black pepper**
- **1 Tsp grated Parmesan cheese**
- **6 cherry tomatoes**
- **7 basil leaves**

DIRECTIONS

1. **Preheat the oven to 400F**
2. **Divide the butter and place it in the oven until is melted.**
3. **Sprinkle the cabbage, basil and the tomatoes and crack two eggs into the ramekins.**
4. **Bake to the desired level of doneness.**

5.   Sprinkle with Parmesan cheese and black pepper.

RATATOUILLE HASH UNDER FRIED EGGS

Serves: **2**
Prep Time: **15**   Minutes

Cook Time: **35**   Minutes

Total Time: **50**   Minutes

INGREDIENTS

- 2 ounces red bell pepper
- 1/8 Tsp salt
- 1/3 cup scallion greens
- 2-ounces zucchini
- ¾ Tsp oregano
- 2-ounces eggplant
- 3 eggs
- 4 Tsp olive oil
- ½ lbs. red potatoes
- 1/8 Tsp black pepper

DIRECTIONS

1. In a skillet heat 2 teaspoons of garlic oil over over medium heat

2. Add potatoes and cook until golden brown for 2-3 minutes

3. Sauté and stir for 1-2 minutes, add eggplant, pepper and salt

4. Cook the vegetables until they are soft for 5 minutes

5. Add oregano, zucchini and cook for 4-5 minutes, add water and stir

6. Remove from heat and stir in the scallions

7. Heat a frying pan and add 1 teaspoon of garlic oil

8. Add eggs into skillet and salt, cook until eggs are ready

Serves: *1*

Prep Time: *15*   Minutes

Cook Time: *10*   Minutes

Total Time: *25*   Minutes

INGREDIENTS

- ¼ cup oats
- ¾ cup coconut milk
- 2 tablespoons coconut flakes
- 2 teaspoons chia seeds
- ½ cup raspberries

DIRECTIONS

1. In a pot whisk oat, coconut milk, salt, raspberries over medium heat
2. Simmer for 10 minutes until oats are tender and add water
3. Pour oatmeal into a bowl with coconut flakes

Serves: *10*
Prep Time: *15*   Minutes

Cook Time: *30*   Minutes

Total Time: *45*   Minutes

INGREDIENTS

- ½ cup pecan halves
- ½ cup butter
- 1/8 teaspoon salt
- 2 teaspoon vanilla extract
- 2 ½ cups rolled oats
- ¼ cup corn syrup
- ½ cup packed brown sugar

DIRECTIONS

1. Preheat oven to 325 F and line a baking dish with parchment
2. Place pecans on a baking sheet and toast for 5-10 minutes
3. Remove from oven and pour in a bowl

4. In a saucepan melt butter over medium heat for 4-5 minutes

5. Stir in brown sugar salt and boil for 1-2 minutes

6. Add oats and pecans to the saucepan and stir, pour the mixture in the baking dish, bake for 15-20 minutes

7. Remove from the oven and let it cook for 10-15 minutes

SPINACH AND QUINOA BREAKFAST

Serves: 8

Prep Time: 25   Minutes

Cook Time: 25   Minutes

Total Time: 50   Minutes

INGREDIENTS

- 1/3 cup quinoa
- 2/3 cup water
- 1/16 teaspoon black pepper
- 2 tablespoons scallion
- 1 ½ ounces bacon

- 4-ounces spinach
- 5 large eggs
- ¼ teaspoon thyme leaves
- 2 pinches sage
- ¼ teaspoon salt
- 2 cups cheddar cheese

DIRECTIONS

1. Preheat oven to 325 F
2. In a saucepan combine quinoa and water and let them boil, after 10-15 minutes remove from heat
3. In a microwave place the frozen spinach and cook for 2-3 minutes
4. In a bowl whisk the eggs and add salt, pepper, scallions, sage and mix with quinoa, bacon and cheese
5. Grease 10 cups of a muffin tin with baking spray and divide the mixture, bake for 20-25 minutes
6. Remove from the oven and let cool them cool before serving

Serves: *4*
Prep Time: *10*   Minutes

Cook Time: *10*   Minutes

Total Time: *10*   Minutes

INGREDIENTS

- 1 lb. ground turkey
- 1 tsp sage
- ½ tsp. salt
- ¼ tsp garlic
- dash white pepper
- dash cayenne pepper
- dash ground nutmeg

DIRECTIONS

1. In a bowl mix all ingredients together
2. Form into patties and cook for 2-3 minutes per side or until golden brown
3. Remove and serve

Serves: *8*
Prep Time: *10*   Minutes

Cook Time: *20*   Minutes

Total Time: *30*   Minutes

INGREDIENTS

- ¼ cup almond flour
- 1 tablespoon coconut flour
- ½ tsp baking soda
- ¼ tsp salt
- 1 egg white
- ¼ tsp coconut oil
- 2 tablespoons water

DIRECTIONS

1. In a bowl mix all dry ingredients
2. In another bowl mix all wet ingredients, add to dry ingredients and mix well
3. Pour mixture into muffin cups and bake at 325 F for 18-20 minutes

4. **Remove and serve with peanut butter or homemade jam**

Serves: *2*

Prep Time: *10* Minutes

Cook Time: *15* Minutes

Total Time: *25* Minutes

INGREDIENTS

- ½ cup low-fat yogurt
- 3 eggs
- 2 cups almond flour
- ¼ tsp salt
- ¼ tsp baking soda
- ½ cup cheddar cheese

DIRECTIONS

1. **Place all ingredients in a blender and blend until smooth**

2. **Pour batter into an electric griddle and cook at 375 F until golden brown on both sides**

3. **Remove on a plate and serve**

BACON AND CHEESE FRITTATAS

Serves: *4*

Prep Time: *10* Minutes

Cook Time: *30* Minutes

Total Time: *40* Minutes

INGREDIENTS

- 3 slices bacon
- 1 cup shredded cheddar
- 6 eggs
- 2 tablespoons water
- ½ tsp salt
- ½ tsp pepper

DIRECTIONS

1. Preheat the oven at 350 F
2. Divide bacon and onion among 8 muffin cups
3. In a bowl whisk eggs and water, salt and pepper
4. Pour over cheese and fill each muffin cup
5. Bake for 20-25 minutes
6. When ready, remove and serve

POTATO LATKES RECIPE

Serves: **4**

Prep Time: **10** Minutes

Cook Time: **30** Minutes

Total Time: **40** Minutes

INGREDIENTS

- ½ cup vegetable oil
- 3 baking potatoes
- 1 egg
- ½ cup flour
- ½ cup onion
- ¼ tsp salt
- ¼ tsp black pepper
- 1 tablespoon parsley

DIRECTIONS

1. In a bowl grate the potatoes and add egg, onion, flour, egg, pepper, salt and mix well
2. In a skillet add 1-2 tablespoons of mixture and cook for 2-3 minutes per side or until golden

3. **When ready, remove and garnish with parsley**

Serves: *4*

Prep Time: *10*   Minutes

Cook Time: *30*   Minutes

Total Time: *40*   Minutes

INGREDIENTS

- 2 tablespoons olive oil
- 1 ground turkey
- ¾ cup diced onion
- 2 tsp garlic
- 2 tablespoon flour
- ¼ cup chicken stock
- ¼ cup rice milk
- 1 tablespoon parsley
- 1 cup mashed potatoes
- ½ tsp paprika

DIRECTIONS

1. Preheat the oven to 375 F

2. In a skillet add olive oil, turkey, garlic and olive oil and sauté for 3-4 minutes

3. Add flour, rice milk, chicken stock and mix well

4. Bring to a boil and simmer for 3-4 minutes

5. Add parsley and place mixture into a casserole dish

6. Bake for 30-35 minutes, sprinkle with paprika and serve

HERBED STUFFING

Serves: *4*
Prep Time: *10*   Minutes

Cook Time: *30*   Minutes

Total Time: *40*   Minutes

INGREDIENTS

-   3 tablespoons olive oil

-   1 cup onions

- 1 clove garlic
- ½ tsp sage
- ½ tsp thyme
- ¾ cup cranberry juice
- ¼ cup chicken stock
- 3 cups stuffing croutons

DIRECTIONS

1. Preheat the oven to 325 F
2. In a skillet add garlic, onions, sage and sauté until soft
3. Add chicken stock, cranberry, croutons and bring to a simmer
4. Transfer to a casserole dish and bake for 18-20 minutes
5. When ready, remove and serve

Serves: *10*
Prep Time: *10*   Minutes

Cook Time: *20*   Minutes

Total Time: *30*   Minutes

INGREDIENTS

- 1 cup water
- 1 package dry active yeast
- 1 cup flour
- 2 tablespoons vegetable oil
- ¼ tsp salt
- 1 cup flour
- 3 cups water
- 2 tablespoons baking soda
- 2 tablespoons salt

DIRECTIONS

1. Preheat the oven to 450 F
2. Dissolve the yeast in a bowl
3. Add flour, salt, vegetable oil and mix well, let the dough rest for 50-60 minutes

4. **Divide into 8-10 balls and roll into pretzel shapes**

5. **Sprinkle with sesame seeds or salt and bake the pretzels for 12-15 minutes**

6. **When ready remove and serve**

Serves: *4*

Prep Time: *10*   Minutes

Cook Time: *15*   Minutes

Total Time: *25*   Minutes

INGREDIENTS

- 1 tablespoon water

- 1 tablespoon Worcestershire sauce

- 1 tsp lemon juice

- 1 tsp mustard

- 3 pork top loin chops

- ¼ tsp lemon seasoning

- 1 tablespoon butter

- 1 tablespoon chives

DIRECTIONS

1. In a bowl add lemon juice, Worcestershire sauce, mustard, mix well and set aside

2. Sprinkle chops with lemon seasoning and place chops in a skillet

3. Cook for 10-12 minutes, transfer to a plate and set aside

4. Pour sauce into skillet and chops over sauce

5. Sprinkle with chives

6. When ready, remove and serve

Serves: *4*

Prep Time: *10*   Minutes

Cook Time: *20*   Minutes

Total Time: *30*   Minutes

INGREDIENTS

- ½ lb. beef
- ½ cup oats
- 2 tablespoons milk
- 1 tsp onion flakes
- ¼ tsp canola oil
- 1 dash pepper

DIRECTIONS

1. In a bowl mix all ingredients and form into patties
2. Heat oil in a skillet and cook each burger for 3-4 minutes per side
3. Remove and serve with potato fries

Serves: *4*
Prep Time: *10*   Minutes

Cook Time: *20*   Minutes

Total Time: *30*   Minutes

INGREDIENTS

- ¾ cup marinade
- 12 oz. chicken breast
- 1 lemon
- 3 wedges

DIRECTIONS

1. In a plastic bag marinade chicken overnight
2. Place chicken on the rack of a broiler pan and broil for 18-20 minutes
3. When ready, serve with lemon or grapes

Serves: *1*

Prep Time: *5*   Minutes

Cook Time: *5*   Minutes

Total Time: *10*   Minutes

INGREDIENTS

- 2 lettuce leaves
- ¾ oz. turkey breast
- 1 tablespoon mayonnaise
- 2 whole crackers
- 5-pieces grapes

DIRECTIONS

1. Cut turkey into small pieces
2. Top lettuce leaves with mayonnaise and turkey
3. Roll lettuce leaves and serve with crackers and grapes

Serves: *6*

Prep Time: *10*   Minutes

Cook Time: *15*   Minutes

Total Time: *25*   Minutes

INGREDIENTS

- ½ cup butter
- 1 tsp thyme
- zest of one orange
- 1 tsp minced garlic
- 2 lbs. shrimp
- ¼ tsp chili powder
- salt

DIRECTIONS

1. In a skillet add thyme leaves and simmer on low heat
2. Remove and add orange zest and cook for 2-3 minutes
3. Add garlic, shrimp, chili powder and cook for 4-5 minutes
4. When ready serve with pasta or rice

Serves: *4*

Prep Time: *10*   Minutes

Cook Time: *20*   Minutes

Total Time: *30*   Minutes

INGREDIENTS

- 1 tablespoon olive oil
- 1 tablespoon butter
- 1 lb. shrimp
- 2 garlic cloves
- 3 tablespoons honey
- 1 tablespoon soy sauce
- 2 tablespoons cilantro

DIRECTIONS

1. In a skillet add garlic, shrimp and cook for 5-6 minutes

2. In another bowl mix soy sauce, cilantro, honey, lime and mix well

3. Add the mixture to the skillet and bring to high heat

4. Cook for 4-5 minutes or until sauce reduces

Serves: *2*

Prep Time: *5*   Minutes

Cook Time: *5*   Minutes

Total Time: *10*   Minutes

INGREDIENTS

- 2 oranges
- 1 grapefruit
- 5 cups baby spinach
- 3 scallions 3 oz. prosciutto

DRESSING

- 2 tablespoons balsamic vinegar
- 2 tablespoons olive oil
- 2 tablespoons cream
- 2 tsp honey
- ½ tsp salt
- ½ tsp black pepper

DIRECTIONS

1. In a bowl mix all ingredients and mix well
2. Serve with dressing

Serves: **2**
Prep Time: **5**   Minutes

Cook Time: **5**   Minutes

Total Time: ***10***   Minutes

INGREDIENTS

- 2 cups cooked pasta
- ½ cup celery
- 2 tablespoons bell pepper
- 2 tablespoons green onion
- 1 tsp lemon zest
- ½ cup low fat mayonnaise
- ½ cup Italian salad dressing
- 4 oz. canned tuna

DIRECTIONS

1. In a bowl mix all ingredients and mix well
2. Serve with dressing

Serves: **2**

Prep Time: **5**   Minutes

Cook Time: **5**   Minutes

Total Time: **10**   Minutes

INGREDIENTS

- **2 cucumber**
- **10 cups salad greens**
- **2 cups sunflower sprouts**
- **2 stalks celery**

DRESSING

- **½ cup lime juice**
- **2 tablespoons fish sauce**
- **¼ tsp honey**
- **1 clove garlic**
- **1 tablespoon cilantro**

DIRECTIONS

1. **In a bowl mix all ingredients and mix well**
2. **Serve with dressing**

Serves: **2**

Prep Time: **5**   Minutes

Cook Time: **5**   Minutes

Total Time: **10**   Minutes

INGREDIENTS

- **3 cups mixed greens**
- **2 mangoes**
- **¼ cucumber**
- **½ cup coconut flakes**
- **1 avocado**

LIME DRESSING

- **½ cup olive oil**
- **1 lime**
- **1 tablespoon apple cider vinegar**
- **½ tsp salt**
- **¼ tsp cinnamon**
- **¼ tsp ginger powder**

DIRECTIONS

1. In a bowl mix all ingredients and mix well

2. Serve with dressing

AVOCADO KALE SALAD

Serves: **2**

Prep Time: **5**   Minutes

Cook Time: **5**   Minutes

Total Time: **10**   Minutes

INGREDIENTS

- 2 cups kale
- 2 tablespoons grapefruit vinaigrette
- 1 tsp salt
- 1 avocado
- 1 grapefruit

DIRECTIONS

1. In a bowl mix all ingredients and mix well

2. Serve with dressing

Serves: **2**

Prep Time: **5**   Minutes

Cook Time: **5**   Minutes

Total Time: **10**   Minutes

INGREDIENTS

- 2 avocados
- 2 tablespoons mayonnaise
- 1 lb. cooked chicken breast
- 3 stalks celery
- ½ Kalamata olives
- 1 tablespoon parsley
- 1 tomato
- salt
- romaine leaves

DIRECTIONS

1. In a bowl mix all ingredients and mix well
2. Serve with dressing

Serves: **2**

Prep Time: **5**   Minutes

Cook Time: **5**   Minutes

Total Time: ***10***   Minutes

INGREDIENTS

- 2 cups broccoli florets
- 2 cups shredded chicken
- 2 handfuls baby spinach
- 2 apples
- ¼ cup raisins
- ½ yellow onion
- ½ cup olive oil
- 1 tablespoon apple cider vinegar
- ¼ tsp salt

DIRECTIONS

1. In a bowl mix all ingredients and mix well
2. Serve with dressing

Serves: **2**

Prep Time: **5**   Minutes

Cook Time: **5**   Minutes

Total Time: **10**   Minutes

INGREDIENTS

- 1 grapefruit
- 1 tablespoon coconut oil
- 1 bunch kale
- 1 tsp salt
- 1 lb. chicken livers
- 1 bunch red beets
- 1 grepefruit
- 1 avocado
- ½ cup mint leaves
- ½ cup balsamic vinegar

DIRECTIONS

1. In a bowl mix all ingredients and mix well
2. Serve with dressing

Serves: **2**
Prep Time: **5**   Minutes

Cook Time: **5**   Minutes

Total Time: **10**   Minutes

INGREDIENTS

- 2 kohlrabi
- 2 tart crisp apples
- 1 bunch watercress

DRESSING

- 1 tablespoon olive oil
- 1 tablespoon apple cider vinegar
- 1 tsp orange blossom water
- 1 tsp honey
- 1 tsp salt

DIRECTIONS

1. In a bowl mix all ingredients and mix well
2. Serve with dressing

Serves: **2**

Prep Time: **5**   Minutes

Cook Time: **5**   Minutes

Total Time: **10**   Minutes

INGREDIENTS

- 1 can sardines
- ½ lb. salad greens
- 2 oz. bacon
- 1 tablespoon olive oil
- 1 tablespoon lemon juice
- salt

DIRECTIONS

1. In a bowl mix all ingredients and mix well
2. Serve with dressing

Serves: *2*

Prep Time: *5*   Minutes

Cook Time: *5*   Minutes

Total Time: *10*   Minutes

INGREDIENTS

- 10 oz. steak
- 4 oz. baby arugula
- 1 lemon
- 1 tsp olive oil
- 1 tsp salt
- black pepper

DIRECTIONS

1. In a bowl mix all ingredients and mix well
2. Serve with dressing

SALMON STEAKS WITH ARUGULA

Serves: *4*

Prep Time: *10*   Minutes

Cook Time: *30*   Minutes

Total Time: *40*   Minutes

INGREDIENTS

- 3 salmon steaks
- canola oil
- 1 tsp black pepper
- 1 cup arugula
- 1 tablespoon capers
- 2 slices lemon

DIRECTIONS

1. Brush salmon with canola oil
2. In a frying pan, fry salmon 3-4 minutes or until golden
3. Remove and serve with pepper and lemon

Serves: *2*
Prep Time: *5*   Minutes

Cook Time: *5*   Minutes

Total Time: *10*   Minutes

INGREDIENTS

- 4 slices bread
- 6 tsp mayonnaise
- 2 slices tomato
- 2 tsp basil
- ¼ tsp salt
- ¼ tsp black pepper

DIRECTIONS

1. Spread mayonnaise over each bread slice
2. Top with basil, tomato slices, pepper, salt and top with bread
3. Serve when ready

Serves: *2*
Prep Time: *10*   Minutes

Cook Time: *25*   Minutes

Total Time: *35*   Minutes

INGREDIENTS

- 1 lb. salmon fillet
- 1 tablespoon dry white wine
- ½ tsp salt
- ground black pepper
- 2 tablespoons shallot
- lemon wedges

DIRECTIONS

1. Preheat the oven to 400 F
2. In a pan place salmon with wine, shallots and pepper
3. Cover and bake for 20-25 minutes
4. When ready, remove and transfer to a plate
5. Serve with lemon wedges

Serves: *2*
Prep Time: *10*   Minutes

Cook Time: *20*   Minutes

Total Time: *30*   Minutes

INGREDIENTS

- 1 gold potato
- 1 tsp olive oil
- ½ tsp salt
- ½ tsp dried thyme

DIRECTIONS

1. Preheat the oven to 425 F
2. Toss potato with salt, thyme and oil
3. Spread potato wedges on a baking sheet
4. Bake for 18-20 minutes or until tender
5. Remove and serve

Serves: *4*

Prep Time: *10*   Minutes

Cook Time: *20*   Minutes

Total Time: *30*   Minutes

INGREDIENTS

- 10 lasagna noodles
- 1 tablespoon olive oil
- 2 cloves garlic
- 1 package tofu
- 2 cups spinach
- ¼ cup Parmesan cheese
- 2 tablespoons Kalamata olives
- ½ tsp red pepper
- ½ tsp salt
- 20 oz. marinara sauce
- ¼ cup mozzarella cheese

DIRECTIONS

1. **In a pot add noodles, water and bring to a boil**

2. **In a skillet add garlic, tofu, spinach and cook for 4-5 minutes**

3. **Transfer to a bowl and stir in red pepper, marinara sauce, Parmesan and olives**

4. **Place a noodle on a cutting board and spread ¼ cup of the tofu filling**

5. **Roll up and place the roll in the pan, repeat with the remaining noodles**

6. **Bring to a simmer and reduce heat on medium for 5-6 minutes, remove when ready**

7. **Sprinkle with mozzarella and serve**

LINGUINE WITH CLAMS

Serves: **4**

Prep Time: **10** Minutes

Cook Time: **20** Minutes

Total Time: **30** Minutes

INGREDIENTS

- 8 oz. linguine pasta

- 1 tablespoon olive oil

- 1 clove garlic

- ½ tsp red pepper

- 28 oz. canned baby clams

- ½ cup dry white wine

- ½ cup chicken broth

- 2 tablespoons parsley

DIRECTIONS

1. Cook pasta according to package indications
2. In a skillet add garlic, red pepper and sauté for 2-3 minutes
3. Add reserved juice, broth, wine and bring to a boil for 5-6 minutes
4. Stir in clams, parsley and toss with pasta
5. Remove from heat and serve

Serves: **6**

Prep Time: **10**   Minutes

Cook Time: **60**   Minutes

Total Time: **70**   Minutes

INGREDIENTS

- 3 tablespoons olive oil
- 1 cup diced onions
- 1//2 cup flour
- 2 cups clam broth
- 1 cup rice milk
- 2 cans chopped clams
- ½ cup tsp white pepper
- 1 tablespoon parsley
- 1 tsp thyme
- 1 bay leaf
- 3 cups potatoes

DIRECTIONS

1. **In a pot sauté onion over medium heat**

2. Add flour, clam broth, rice milk and whisk until smooth

3. Add white pepper, parsley, thyme clams, bay leaf and bring to a boil

4. Cook for 40 minutes, add diced potatoes and simmer for 15-20 minutes

5. Remove from heat and serve

Serves: *4*

Prep Time: *10*   Minutes

Cook Time: *20*   Minutes

Total Time: *30*   Minutes

INGREDIENTS

- 10 oz. shrimp
- ½ cup olive oil
- 1 tsp garlic
- 1 tablespoon shallots
- ¼ cup tomato

- ¼ cup white wine
- ½ cup lemon juice
- 1 tablespoon parsley
- 3 cups linguine

DIRECTIONS

1. In a skillet add shrimp and sauté for 2-3 minutes
2. Remove and set aside
3. Add shallots, tomato, garlic, lemon juice, wine and bring to a boil
4. Reduce heat and simmer for 5-6 minutes
5. Add linguine, shrimp, parsley to the skillet and toss the pasta in the sauce
6. Cook until done, remove from heat and serve

TURKEY BURGERS

Serves: **4**

Prep Time: **10** Minutes

Cook Time: **30** Minutes

Total Time: **40** Minutes

INGREDIENTS

- 1 lb. ground turkey
- 2 tablespoons olive oil
- 1 tablespoon onion flakes
- ½ tsp garlic powder
- ½ tsp oregano
- 1 tablespoon parsley
- ¼ tsp salt

DIRECTIONS

1. In a bowl place turkey, onion flakes, olive oil, garlic powder, salt, parsley and oregano
2. Mix well and divide into 4-6 thin patty shapes
3. Place on a tray and refrigerate
4. Preheat grill
5. Place the turkey burgers on the grill and cook for 4-5 minutes per side
6. When ready, remove and serve with potato wedges

Serves: **2**

Prep Time: **5**   Minutes

Cook Time: **5**   Minutes

Total Time: **10**   Minutes

INGREDIENTS

- **2 cups vegetable juice**
- **2 tablespoons lime juice**
- **1 tsp Worcestershire sauce**
- **¼ tsp horseradish**
- **1 cup ice cubes**
- **1 cup hot pepper sauce**

DIRECTIONS

1. **In a pitcher add vegetable juice, lime, Worcestershire juice, hot pepper sauce and horseradish**
2. **Garnish with celery and serve**

Serves: **4**

Prep Time: **10** Minutes

Cook Time: **30** Minutes

Total Time: **40** Minutes

INGREDIENTS

- 2 sweet potatoes
- 3 cups vegetable broth
- ¼ cup onion
- 1 cup kale
- 1 tsp paprika
- 1 tsp garlic powder
- ¼ tsp ginger
- 1 tablespoon olive oil
- 1 tsp salt

DIRECTIONS

1. Preheat the oven to 350 F
2. Microwave sweet potatoes for 10-12 minutes, then bake for 20 minutes
3. Remove from the oven and place them in a blender

4. Add the rest of ingredients and blend until smooth

5. Transfer soup to a soup pot and cook on low heat

6. Add kale leaves and simmer until ready to serve

SWISS CHARD & SWEET POTATO SOUP

Serves: **4**

Prep Time: **10** Minutes

Cook Time: **30** Minutes

Total Time: **40** Minutes

INGREDIENTS

- 1 cup duck fat
- 1 onion
- 1,5 lbs. zucchini
- 1 oz. sweet potato
- 3 cups bone broth
- 1 Swiss chard
- 1 bunch cilantro
- ½ lemon juice

DIRECTIONS

1. In a saucepan add onions and sauté for 10 minutes
2. Add sweet potato, zucchini and stir to coat
3. Add bone broth and the rest of ingredients and cook on low heat until potato is soft
4. Pure soup until smooth
5. Return soup to the saucepan and cook until ready to serve

BLUEBERRY SOUP

Serves: **4**
Prep Time: **10**   Minutes

Cook Time: **60**   Minutes

Total Time: **70**   Minutes

INGREDIENTS

-   2 cups blueberries
-   1 can coconut milk
-   ¼ tsp rosemary

-   ½ tsp cinnamon

-   1 tablespoon apple cider vinegar

-   1 tablespoon lemon juice

-   1 pinch salt

DIRECTIONS

1. In a pot add all ingredients and cook for 10-12 minutes
2. Allow to cook for 30 minutes
3. Pour soup in a blender and blend until smooth
4. Pour in a bowl and garnish with rosemary

HOMEMADE THAI CHICKEN BROTH

Serves: *8*
Prep Time: *10*   Minutes

Cook Time: *10*   Minutes

Total Time: *20*   Minutes

INGREDIENTS

- 1 chicken
- 1 stalk lemongrass
- 16-18 basil leaves
- 4 slices ginger
- 1 lime
- 1 tsp salt

DIRECTIONS

1. In a slow cooker add chicken, lemon grass, basil leaves and cook on low for 8-10 hours
2. Ladle the broth into a bowl, add salt, lime juice and garnish basil leaves
3. Serve when ready

LEEK AND CAULIFLOWER SOUP WITH BACON

Serves: *4*

Prep Time: *10*   Minutes

Cook Time: *30*   Minutes

Total Time: *40*   Minutes

INGREDIENTS

-   1 leek
-   1 onion
-   1 cauliflower
-   1 tablespoon coconut oil
-   2 lbs. chicken broth

DIRECTIONS

1. In a pot sauté onion and leek for 4-5 minutes
2. Add cauliflower, chicken broth and broil to a boil, simmer for 10-12 minutes
3. Pure the soup, garnish with bacon bits and serve

BASIL SOUP

Serves: *4*
Prep Time: *10*   Minutes

Cook Time: *30*   Minutes

Total Time: *40*   Minutes

INGREDIENTS

- 2 tablespoons butter
- ¼ onion
- 1 carrot
- 1 lb. blanched tomatoes
- 2 cup homemade chicken
- 2 tablespoons dried basil
- ¼ tsp salt
- ¼ tsp pepper

DIRECTIONS

1. In a saucepan met butter, add carrot, onion and sauté for 4-5 minutes
2. Add beef broth, tomatoes, salt, basil and simmer for 15-20 minutes
3. Cool and blend mixture until smooth
4. Pour into bowls and serve

Serves: *4*

Prep Time: *10*   Minutes

Cook Time: *35*   Minutes

Total Time: *45*   Minutes

INGREDIENTS

- **2-quarts turkey stock**
- **2 beets**
- **1 onion**
- **3 carrots**
- **2 cups peas**
- **2 cups green beans**
- **¼ head cabbage**
- **8 Swiss chard leaves**
- **2 cups cooked turkey meat**

DIRECTIONS

1. **In a pot add turkey stock, beets, greens, onions and cook over medium heat**

2. **Add carrots, peas, green beans, cabbage, Swiss chars leaves and bring to boil**

3. Simmer for about 30 minutes, add turkey meat and
    simmer for another 5-10 minutes

4. Remove from heat and serve

CAULIFLOWER SOUP

Serves:	**4**	
Prep Time:	**10**	Minutes
Cook Time:	**30**	Minutes
Total Time:	**40**	Minutes

INGREDIENTS

-   ½ onion
-   2 tablespoons coconut
-   1-quart chicken stock
-   1-quart water
-   1 head cauliflower
-   5 sausages
-   2 cups coconut milk
-   2 tablespoons minced garlic

- 1 tablespoon oregano
- ¼ tablespoon sage
- ½ tablespoon paprika
- salt

DIRECTIONS

1. In a pot add onion, oil and sauté over medium heat for 8-10 minutes
2. Add cauliflower to the pot, cover with stock and water and bring to boil
3. Cook until cauliflower is tender and add sausage and remaining ingredients
4. When ready remove from heat and serve

RICE SOUP

Serves: *4*
Prep Time: *10*   Minutes

Cook Time: *30*   Minutes

Total Time: *40*   Minutes

INGREDIENTS

- 1 cup onion
- 1 cup celery
- 1 cup baby carrot
- 1 tablespoon olive oil
- 1/3 cup white rice
- black pepper
- 3 thyme springs
- 1 bay leaf
- 10 cups no-salt chicken broth
- 2 cooked chicken breasts
- 2 tablespoons lime juice

DIRECTIONS

1. In a soup pot add all soup ingredients
2. Sauté for 5-6 minutes
3. Add water simmer for 20-30 minutes
4. Season with pepper
5. When ready, pour into bowls and serve

Serves: **4**

Prep Time: **10**   Minutes

Cook Time: **10**   Minutes

Total Time: **20**   Minutes

INGREDIENTS

- 1 avocado
- 2 romaine lettuce leaves
- 1 cup coconut milk
- 1 tablespoon lime juice
- 16-18 mint leaves
- salt

DIRECTIONS

1. Place all ingredients in a blender and blend until smooth
2. Pour in a bowl and place in the fridge for 10-15 before serving

LEMON CHEESECAKES

Serves: *10*

Prep Time: *20* Minutes

Cook Time: *20* Minutes

Total Time: *40* Minutes

INGREDIENTS

- 1 cup yogurt
- 5 oz. cookies
- ½ cup sliced almonds
- 2 tablespoons butter
- 2 cups cottage cheese
- 2 tablespoons cornstarch
- 2/3 cup sugar
- 3 eggs
- 2 tablespoons lemon zest
- 2 tablespoons lemon juice
- 1 teaspoon vanilla extract

DIRECTIONS

1. Preheat oven to 300 F and line a 12 cup muffin tin with baking liners

2. In a blender add almonds and cookies and blend

3. Melt butter on high heat for 1-2 minutes and pour the crumb into the melted butter,

4. Press the crumbs on the bottom of the cups

5. Use again the blender and add cottage cheese, yogurt, cornstarch, and blend for 1-2 minutes, add sugar, lemon juice, vanilla extract and eggs and blend for 1-2 minutes

6. Pour the mixture into muffin cups, bake for 25-30 minutes

7. Remove from the oven let them cool and serve!

BUCKWHEAT WAFFLES

Serves: *4*

Prep Time: *10*   Minutes

Cook Time: *20*   Minutes

Total Time: *30*   Minutes

INGREDIENTS

- 3 teaspoons butter
- ½ cup sugar
- 3 eggs
- 1/3 cup lime juice
- 2 cup almond milk
- 2 tablespoons cider vinegar
- 1 tablespoons canola oil
- ½ teaspoon vanilla extract
- ½ teaspoon almond extract
- 2 cups rice flour
- ¾ cup buckwheat flour
- ½ teaspoon salt
- 3 tablespoons brown sugar
- 1 ½ teaspoons baking powder
- ¼ teaspoons nutmeg
- 1/8 teaspoon cardamom

DIRECTIONS

1. In a saucepan melt butter over medium heat
2. In a bowl beat an egg and whisk with lime juice, stir constantly and heat the mixture over low heat
3. In a blender beat milk, egg, vinegar, vanilla extract, oil and almond milk
4. In another bowl stir rice flour, brown sugar, baking powder, buckwheat flour, salt, nutmeg and cardamom, add the flour mixture and beat until smooth

5. Brush an iron oil with oil and pour some mixture into the waffle iron and cook for 5-6 minutes

6. Remove and serve!

SALMON CAKES

Serves: **6**

Prep Time: **15** Minutes

Cook Time: **10** Minutes

Total Time: **25** Minutes

INGREDIENTS

- 1 teaspoons mayonnaise
- 2 teaspoon garlic oil
- 1 ½ teaspoons lemon juice
- ¼ teaspoon black pepper
- ¼ cup bread crumbs
- 2 tablespoons olive oil
- 3 lemon wedges
- 2 teaspoons fresh dill

- 14-ounce can salmon

- 1 egg

- ¼ chopped celery

- ¼ cup sliced scallion greens

- ½ cup oats

- 2 tablespoons tomato paste

DIRECTIONS

1. For aioli, in a bowl stir mayonnaise, garlic oil, lemon juice and chopped dill, cover and chill

2. For the fish cakes mash the salmon in a bowl and stir in egg, oats, tomato paste scallion greens and pepper, cover and chill

3. In a skillet heat oil over medium heat and fry cakes for 4-5 minutes each side

4. Garnish them with a dollop of sauce and dill

Serves: *10*

Prep Time: *10*   Minutes

Cook Time: *40*   Minutes

Total Time: *50*   Minutes

INGREDIENTS

- 2 eggs
- 1 ¼ cup whole milk
- ½ cup maple syrup
- 3 tablespoons rice flour
- 1 tablespoons cornstarch
- 2 tablespoons tapioca flour
- 2 teaspoon vinegar
- 5 tablespoons butter
- 1 teaspoons vanilla extract
- 2 ¼ dried coconut

DIRECTIONS

1. Preheat the oven to 350 F and place a rack into it and butter a pie plate

2. In a bowl mix milk, maple syrup, eggs and whisk, stir
    in cornstarch, vinegar, tapioca flour, rice flour, melted
    butter, vanilla and coconut flakes

3. Pour the mixture into a pie plate, bake for 40-45
    minutes, let it chill for a couple of hours and sprinkle
    with sugar

CHOCOLATE HAZELNUT BITES

Serves: **12**

Prep Time: **15**   Minutes

Cook Time: **0**   Minutes

Total Time: **15**   Minutes

INGREDIENTS

-   2 cups rolled oats
-   ¼ Tsp salt
-   1 Tsp sugar
-   2 Tsp canola oil
-   2 Tsp vanilla extract
-   1/3 cup brown sugar

- ¼ cup water

- 2 Tsp chia seeds

- ¾ cup hazelnuts

- 1 Tsp peanut butter

- ¼ cup sifted sorghum flour

- ¼ cup unsweetened cocoa powder

DIRECTIONS

1. Mix water and brown sugar in a saucepan over medium heat, stir for 2-3 minutes
2. Add canola oil, peanut butter and reduce heat
3. In a food processor add sorghum flour, cocoa, oats, salt and chia seeds and blend
4. Pour the mixture in the brown sugar and mix for 1 minute
5. Place them on a baking sheet with waxed pepper and put in the refrigerator for 60-90 minutes

Serves: *2*
Prep Time: *10*   Minutes

Cook Time: *10*   Minutes

Total Time: *20*   Minutes

INGREDIENTS

- 1 orange
- ½ cup organic mayonnaise
- 1 cup grapes
- 1 apples
- 1 banana
- ½ cup unsweetened coconut
- ½ cup pecans
- ½ cup cherries
- ½ cup raisins

DIRECTIONS

1. In a bowl mix mayonnaise and orange juice
2. In another bowl mix all salad ingredients and divide into 2-3 bowls
3. Drizzle mayonnaise mixture and serve

Serves: **4**
Prep Time: **10** Minutes

Cook Time: **10** Minutes

Total Time: **20** Minutes

INGREDIENTS

- 1 cup almond flour
- 3 eggs
- 3 tablespoons honey
- 2 tablespoons vanilla
- ½ tsp salt
- ½ tsp baking soda
- 1 tablespoon butter
- homemade jam

DIRECTIONS

1. In a blender mix all ingredients and blend until smooth
2. Pour batter into an electric griddle and cook at 275 degrees
3. Cook until until golden brown, serve with jam

Serves: **2**

Prep Time: **10**   Minutes

Cook Time: **10**   Minutes

Total Time: **20**   Minutes

INGREDIENTS

- **2 cups blueberries**
- **¼ cup honey**

DIRECTIONS

1. **In a saucepan add frozen blueberries and honey**
2. **Boil for 10-12 minutes, until blueberries are soft**
3. **Pour in a bowl and serve**

Serves: *4*

Prep Time: *10*   Minutes

Cook Time: *10*   Minutes

Total Time: *20*   Minutes

INGREDIENTS

- ½ cup cooked quinoa
- ½ cup peanut butter
- 1 tablespoon chia seeds
- ½ tsp vanilla
- ¼ tablespoon maple syrup

DIRECTIONS

1. In a bowl mix peanut butter and quinoa
2. Add maple syrup, vanilla and chia seeds
3. Roll mixture into balls and store in the refrigerator

Serves: **2**

Prep Time: **10**   Minutes

Cook Time: **10**   Minutes

Total Time: **20**   Minutes

INGREDIENTS

- 1 banana
- ½ tablespoon peanut butter
- ½ tsp chia seeds
- ½ tsp shredded coconut

DIRECTIONS

1. Slice a banana in half, lengthwise
2. Spread each slice with peanut butter and sprinkle with shredded coconut and chia seeds
3. Serve when ready

Serves: *1*

Prep Time: *5*   Minutes

Cook Time: *5*   Minutes

Total Time: *10*   Minutes

INGREDIENTS

- 12 chai tea ice cubes
- 2 cups milk
- 1 tablespoon maple syrup
- chocolate syrup
- whipped cream

DIRECTIONS

1. In a blender place all ingredients and blend until smooth
2. Pour smoothie in a glass and serve

Serves: *1*

Prep Time: *5* Minutes

Cook Time: *5* Minutes

Total Time: *10* Minutes

INGREDIENTS

- 10 pitted dates
- ½ cup almonds
- 1 tablespoon cacao powder
- 1 tsp instant coffee
- ¼ cup almond breeze
- 5 ice cubes

DIRECTIONS

1. In a blender place all ingredients and blend until smooth
2. Pour smoothie in a glass and serve

Serves: *1*

Prep Time: **5** Minutes

Cook Time: **5** Minutes

Total Time: **10** Minutes

INGREDIENTS

- 2 bananas
- 5 ice cubes
- 1 tablespoon coconut oil
- 1 tablespoon diary free yogurt
- 1 tablespoon chia seeds
- 1 tablespoon hemp seeds
- 1 tsp camu powder
- 1 tablespoon cocoa
- ½ cup coconut milk

DIRECTIONS

1. In a blender place all ingredients and blend until smooth

2. Pour smoothie in a glass and serve

Serves: *1*
Prep Time: **5**   Minutes

Cook Time: **5**   Minutes

Total Time: **10**   Minutes

INGREDIENTS

- 10 oz. frozen raspberries
- ¼ cup vanilla kefir
- 1 tablespoon hemp
- 1 cup orange juice

DIRECTIONS

1. **In a blender place all ingredients and blend until smooth**
2. **Pour smoothie in a glass and serve**

Serves: *1*

Prep Time: *5*   Minutes

Cook Time: *5*   Minutes

Total Time: *10*   Minutes

INGREDIENTS

- 1 cup ice
- 1/3 cup peaches
- 1 tsp sugar
- 2 tablespoons powdered egg whites

DIRECTIONS

1. In a blender place all ingredients and blend until smooth
2. Pour smoothie in a glass and serve

Serves: *1*

Prep Time: *5*   Minutes

Cook Time: *5*   Minutes

Total Time: *10*   Minutes

INGREDIENTS

- 1 orange
- 1 squeeze of lime
- 1 bunch of cilantro
- ¼ cup pineapple
- 1 stalk asparagus

DIRECTIONS

1. In a blender place all ingredients and blend until smooth
2. Pour smoothie in a glass and serve

Serves: *1*

Prep Time: *5*   Minutes

Cook Time: *5*   Minutes

Total Time: *10*   Minutes

INGREDIENTS

- ½ cup pasteurized liquid egg product
- ¼ cup non-dairy whipped topping
- almond extract
- ½ cup berries
- vanilla extract

DIRECTIONS

1. In a blender place all ingredients and blend until smooth
2. Pour smoothie in a glass and serve

Serves: *1*

Prep Time: *5* Minutes

Cook Time: *5* Minutes

Total Time: *10* Minutes

INGREDIENTS

- 6 oz. water
- 1 cup pineapple
- 1 orange
- 1 carrot
- 1 tablespoon chia seeds
- ½ tsp ginger
- 1 handful baby spinach

DIRECTIONS

1. In a blender place all ingredients and blend until smooth
2. Pour smoothie in a glass and serve

Serves: *1*

Prep Time: **5**   Minutes

Cook Time: **5**   Minutes

Total Time: *10*   Minutes

INGREDIENTS

- 4 oz. water
- 1 mango
- 1 kiwifruit
- 1 cup kale

DIRECTIONS

1. **In a blender place all ingredients and blend until smooth**
2. **Pour smoothie in a glass and serve**

Serves: *1*

Prep Time: *5*   Minutes

Cook Time: *5*   Minutes

Total Time: *10*   Minutes

INGREDIENTS

- 5 oz. water
- 1 banana
- 3 strawberries
- 1 orange
- 1 baby spinach

DIRECTIONS

1. In a blender place all ingredients and blend until smooth
2. Pour smoothie in a glass and serve

Serves: *1*

Prep Time: *5*   Minutes

Cook Time: *5*   Minutes

Total Time: *10*   Minutes

INGREDIENTS

- 2 tsp Matcha
- ¼ cup spinach
- ½ avocado
- ½ banana
- ½ cup coconut water
- ½ cup orange juice

DIRECTIONS

1. **In a blender place all ingredients and blend until smooth**
2. **Pour smoothie in a glass and serve**

Serves: *1*
Prep Time: *5*   Minutes

Cook Time: *5*   Minutes

Total Time: *10*   Minutes

INGREDIENTS

- 1 green apple
- 3 cups spinach
- 1 cup ice cubes
- ¼ cup water
- 1 tsp lemon juice

DIRECTIONS

1. In a blender place all ingredients and blend until smooth
2. Pour smoothie in a glass and serve

Serves: *1*

Prep Time: *5* Minutes

Cook Time: *5* Minutes

Total Time: *10* Minutes

INGREDIENTS

- 1 tsp matcha
- 1 tsp water
- ½ cup strawberries
- ½ cup blueberries
- ½ banana
- ¼ cup orange juice

DIRECTIONS

1. In a blender place all ingredients and blend until smooth
2. Pour smoothie in a glass and serve